CAREERS IN NUTRITION

DIETITIAN

NUTRITIONIST

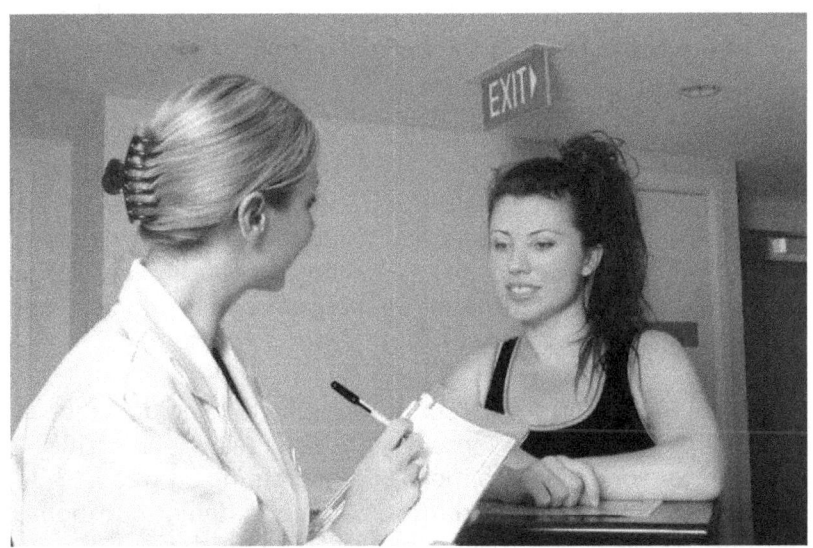

NUTRITIONISTS AND DIETITIANS PROVIDE guidance on how to improve human health through nutrition. They study the effects of nutrition, and devise strategies for eating practices that promote wellness, and prevent or treat disease.

While the terms "nutritionist" and "dietitian" are often used interchangeably, the American Dietetic Association rules that a practitioner can only use the title dietitian after meeting strict, specific educational and experience prerequisites and passing a national registration examination. The title nutritionist, on the other hand, is protected by some but not all states. This means that in some areas anyone can use the title nutritionist, regardless of education and training.

The standard education path for nutritionists and dietitians is to complete a bachelor's degree in dietetics, foods and nutrition, food service systems management, or other related areas. Passing a licensure exam is required in many states. To obtain certification, students must complete a one-year supervised internship and pass an exam, in addition to the bachelor's degree. Master's and PhD programs are also available. These are necessary for those who want to teach at the university level, or to work in advanced clinical positions.

There is a variety of different work settings and duties available for nutritionists and dietitians. Many work in hospitals and other healthcare facilities alongside physicians. Others provide nutritional counseling for groups or individuals. Some go into marketing. Because there are so many different nutritional philosophies, nutritionists and dietitians can vary greatly from person to person.

There is an enormous amount of research being done about all types of nutrition these days, which makes it an exciting field to work in. It also means the job outlook is good. Growing awareness of nutrition, and of different nutritional philosophies, has broadened the field of nutrition and increased the number of jobs. This interest is expected to continue.

Working conditions for nutritionists and dietitians are generally good and so is the pay. The average annual salary of a nutritionist is $50,000, and the top earners can make more than $75,000. Those with graduate degrees can expect to earn higher salaries. Generally speaking, nutritionists and dietitians working in education and research earn the most out of all the different types of nutrition-based careers.

Most nutritionists and dietitians are drawn to this field of work because they are passionate about helping people achieve optimal health. Their work is a great gift. Although they aren't saving lives on a daily basis like emergency room doctors, nutritionists and dietitians have a profound, life-long influence on well-being. If you are passionate about food and its effects on the body, read on. This could be a fulfilling career for you.

WHAT YOU CAN DO NOW

A CAREER IN NUTRITION TYPICALLY requires a college education so your focus in high school will be preparation for college entrance requirements. This usually means four years each of English, math, and sciences. Chemistry and biology are a must. If your school offers courses in microbiology, physiology, or nutrition, you should definitely take them. They will look good on your college application, and will give you a head start for studying nutrition in college.

Being a nutritionist isn't all about science though. It is a good idea to take courses in communications, psychology, sociology, statistics, and economics. These will provide insight into the marketing and interpersonal aspects of the nutrition field.

Ask your science teacher or guidance counselor for assistance in finding a nutritionist or dietitian in your area you can talk to. Hospitals and public health clinics are a great place to start. When speaking with nutritionists, be sure to ask questions such as what they like and dislike about their jobs, what their daily routine is like, where they went to school, and what advice they have for a prospective nutrition student. Talk to as many different nutritionists and dietitians as you can. This will give you a good idea of the various types of work that are available.

Spend some time researching the field. Look for nutrition magazines, journals, and books at your local library. Check out the American Dietetic Association at www.eatright.org. They have great resources for students as well as health professionals in the nutrition field. The American Nutrition Association also has information, including online newsletters.

HISTORY OF THE PROFESSION

THE STUDY OF NUTRITION SEEMS LIKE a recent phenomenon, but it has actually been going on since ancient times. As early as 475 BC, the Greek philosopher Anaxagoras stated that nutrients needed to sustain and reproduce life were contained in foods. Not long after that observation, the Greek physician Hippocrates said, "Let thy food be thy medicine and thy medicine be thy food." Hippocrates had the same viewpoint as nutritionists and dietitians today: that food can be used to maintain wellness, and prevent and even treat illness. In fact, foods were often used as medicines in ancient Greece.

One of the first recorded nutritional experiments is in the Bible's Book of Daniel. The book tells the story of Daniel and his friends when they were captured by the king of Babylon during an invasion of Israel. They were selected as court servants and invited to eat and drink from the king's supply of fine foods and wines. However, they opted to eat vegetables and water in accordance with their Jewish dietary restrictions. The king's chief steward allowed them to follow their own diet for 10 days, after which they were compared to the king's men. Daniel and his friends appeared healthier, and were allowed to continue with their diet.

The first scientific nutrition experiment was conducted in 1747. Dr. James Lind, a physician in the British navy, observed that sailors on long journeys were developing scurvy, a deadly bleeding disorder. The sailors were only eating bread and meat; no fruits or vegetables. Dr. Lind experimented by giving one group of soldiers salt water, one group vinegar, and one group limes. Those who were given limes did not develop scurvy. The discovery was largely ignored for many years, and it wasn't until the 1930s that Vitamin C – the key nutrient in the lime juice – was identified. Afterwards, British sailors were commonly called "Limeys."

New developments in the study of nutrition arose during the Enlightenment and Victorian Ages. For example, Antoine Lavoisier, the "Father of Nutrition and Chemistry," discovered the process by which food is metabolized. In 1770, he demonstrated that the oxidation of food is the source of body heat and energy.

In the early 1800s, scientists recognized that the elements oxygen, nitrogen, hydrogen, and carbon are the primary components of food. Soon after, methods were developed to measure the proportions of the elements, and their connections with health. Francois Magendie identified protein as an essential dietary component in 1816. He had observed that dogs fed only carbohydrates and fat lost their body protein, and died within a few weeks, but dogs who were also fed protein survived.

The actual chemical makeup of carbohydrates, fats, and proteins were discovered by Justus Liebig, a pioneer in early plant growth studies, in 1840. Twenty years later, Claude Bernard proved that body fat can be synthesized from carbohydrate and protein, in other words, that the energy in blood glucose can be stored as fat.

Another important health experiment with sailors occurred in the 1880s, when Kanehiro Takaki observed that Japanese sailors developed a disease called beriberi, which causes heart problems and paralysis, while Japanese naval officers and British sailors did not. When the Japanese sailors added vegetables and meats to their diets, the disease rates plummeted.

Similarly, in 1897, a Dutchman named Christiaan Eijkman observed that some of the natives of Java fell sick with beriberi. He experimented on chickens and found that when chickens were fed the native diet of white rice, they developed the symptoms of beriberi. When he fed them unprocessed brown rice with the outer bran intact, the chickens did not develop the disease. Eijkman tried feeding brown rice to his patients, and they were cured. Nutritionists later learned that the outer rice bran contains the Vitamin B1, or thiamine.

Dietetics and nutrition became a recognized profession near the end of the 19th century, when trained nutritionists began working in American hospitals. In 1912, E. V. McCollum, a US Department of Agriculture researcher at the University of Wisconsin, used a new approach to the study of nutrition that linked certain diseases to specific vitamin deficiencies. It was in that same year that a Polish doctor named Casimir Funk coined the term "vitamine" to describe the essential factors in the diet. The term was derived from two words: "vital," because vitamins are required for life, and "amine," because vitamins were originally thought to be amines, compounds derived from ammonia.

Many vitamins were discovered and isolated in the early 20th century. During this time, supplemental vitamins made an appearance and the marketing of the first vitamin pills created a new industry around science-based health products.

The first Recommended Dietary Allowances (RDAs) were established by the National Research Council in 1941. In the early 1950s, USDA nutritionists made a new set of guidelines that also included the number of servings of each food group in order to make it easier for people to receive their RDAs of each nutrient. The RDAs have subsequently been revised every five to 10 years. Although RDAs are still being used in nutrition labeling of foods, a new system of nutrition recommendations was introduced in 1997. The Dietary Reference Intake (DRI) was developed by the Institute of Medicine of the US National Academy of

Sciences. It is intended for the general public, but used mostly by health professionals when preparing institutional diets or helping industries develop new food stuffs. It is also used by public health officials when making healthcare policy changes.

The US Department of Agriculture (USDA) introduced the food guide pyramid in 1992. The original American pyramid was divided into six horizontal sections, with each section containing a depiction of foods from that food group. For example, the biggest, bottom section, was labeled the "Bread, Cereal, Rice, and Pasta Group," and had pictures of loaves of bread, a plate of pasta, a bowl of cereal, a bowl of rice, and a few crackers.

The food pyramid was updated in 2005 and renamed "MyPyramid." It replaced the original horizontal sections with colorful vertical wedges. It also featured a figure walking up the side of the pyramid to represent the importance of exercise. The MyPyramid was not popular because it was too hard to figure out how much food each wedge actually represented. To solve the problem, the USDA introduced the new "MyPlate" program in June 2011. MyPlate was designed to visually define how many fruits, vegetables, grains, and proteins should be on our plates at meal time. It is simple enough to follow that even school children can easily understand it.

In 1994 Congress approved the Dietary and Supplement Health and Education Act. The act establishes what can and cannot be said about nutritional supplements without prior Food and Drug Administration (FDA) review. This is why many vitamin bottle labels include a disclaimer stating that their products and information are not intended to diagnose, cure, or prevent any disease. In January of 2000, the FDA altered the 1994 act by allowing supplement makers to state that their products can improve the structure or function of the body, or improve common minor symptoms. Since then, the labels on vitamin, herb, and nutrient products often list statements such as "strengthens joint structure," "helps you relax," or "maintains a healthy heart."

The fields of nutrition and alternative medicine have experienced tremendous growth in recent years. More and more people are supplementing or even substituting their traditional medical care with alternative nutrition-based treatments. Magazines, TV shows, Internet sites, and newspapers have increased the number of articles discussing nutrition and its effects on health. While not all Americans have good nutrition, few can claim they are unaware that it affects their health and well-being.

WHERE YOU WILL WORK

DIETITIANS AND NUTRITIONISTS work in many different settings. The biggest employers are hospitals, nursing care facilities, outpatient care centers, and offices of physicians or other healthcare professionals. Many dietitians and nutritionists can be found working in schools, prisons, community health centers, supermarkets, health clubs, and marketing firms.

Sports and health clubs often employ nutritionists and dietitians to consult with clients about how nutrition affects athletic performance, or even just general fitness. These nutritionists and dietitians usually come into work for appointments rather than staying there all day. They consult with clients onsite in an office, and may even walk around the health club with the client to observe the individual's workout routine.

Supermarkets and advertising firms employ nutritionists and dietitians to help them market certain products. In this case, the work site is typically an office setting, removed from the actual food production and sales. They may work alongside managers, consultants, and market analysts.

In a sense, all nutritionists and dietitians are teachers, even if they are only teaching one individual at a time. Some choose to teach in the classic sense – in the classroom. There are opportunities to teach diet and nutrition at every level – elementary and middle schools, high schools, and of course, colleges and universities. Those teaching basic or theoretical nutrition in elementary, middle, or high school can expect to work in the same standard classrooms used for teaching most subjects. At the college level, instruction is still provided in classroom settings, but laboratory work is often part of the curriculum. This may include chemical experiments in college laboratories, or behavioral experiments that can take place anywhere it is possible to monitor people's eating habits.

For the most part, dietitians and nutritionists work in clean, light, and well-ventilated facilities. All healthcare facilities are required to abide by certain standards of cleanliness. So are schools and prisons, although these may have lower standards than healthcare facilities. The situation isn't quite so pleasant for nutritionists and dietitians in food management, who often work in hot, congested kitchens.

Many professionals in this field prefer to go into private practice. Depending on how ambitious or successful they are, these practitioners may have offices that include several rooms or an entire floor of an office building. In any case, the rooms are designed to be relaxing. There is typically soft lighting, comfortable chairs, and attractive décor such as contemporary artwork on the walls. The goal is to make clients feel as comfortable as possible when talking about nutrition. However, when private practices include on-site medical testing, they often look more like a healthcare facility, with bright lighting, examination tables, and medical instruments.

The majority of dietitians and nutritionists work a standard 40-hour workweek. However, some of those hours may include weekends. This is usually the case when a healthcare facility requires it, or if the professional is part of a private practice catering to clients who want weekend appointments.

THE WORK YOU WILL DO

NUTRITIONISTS AND DIETICIANS ARE employed to promote healthy eating in a variety of different settings and for a variety of different purposes. They study how nutrition affects health, disease and behavior. They use their knowledge of nutrition to help schools, corporations, hospitals, and individuals to achieve a better state of wellness through dietary changes and eating habits.

Common job duties of dieticians and nutritionists are the planning of food and nutrition programs, the supervision of meal preparation, and the overseeing of the serving of meals. They manage food service systems for institutions such as hospitals, schools, and prisons. By promoting healthy eating habits and recommending dietary modifications, dieticians help prevent and treat illnesses.

There are many different schools of thought in the nutrition world. Some people believe in alternative diets such as vegetarianism, veganism, and the raw food diet, to name a few. Others believe that a diet following the United States Department of Agriculture's (USDA) food pyramid is the way to go. Most nutritionists and dieticians follow a certain line of thought and stick to it in their work. Nonetheless, they remain aware of the other ideas and principles in practice. They need that knowledge to expand upon their own thinking and to be able to advocate their philosophy in a well-informed manner.

New research is constantly coming out about nutrition and how it affects our lives. Nutritionists are often at the forefront of this research. Some research is generalized, while other times it focuses on a particular test study. Keeping up with all the research in the nutrition field is an important part of this career.

Clinical Dietitians

There are a number of different types of dieticians and nutritionists. Clinical dieticians work in hospitals, nursing care facilities, and other medical institutions. The primary job duties of clinical dieticians are to assess the nutritional needs of patients, to develop and implement corresponding nutrition programs, and then evaluate and report the results. They regularly consult with doctors and other healthcare professionals.

Some clinical dieticians specialize in certain areas. They may concentrate on helping overweight patients manage their weight. Or they may specialize in the care of patients with renal (kidney) problems, diabetes, eating disorders, or those who are critically ill. Clinical dieticians may also manage the food service department in correctional facilities, small hospitals, or nursing care facilities.

On a regular work day, these are the duties a clinical dietician may perform:

Meet with physicians to discuss the medical condition of new patients.

Meet with new patients for an initial consultation. Ask questions about eating habits and nutritional history. Develop an eating plan for new patients based on their medical needs.

Visit current patients to evaluate how their eating programs are going and to assess their nutritional health. This may involve weighing the patient.

Write up reports about the patients' conditions for future reference and for the doctor's use.

Read books and articles on nutrition, especially how medical conditions affect nutrition needs. It is essential that clinical dieticians understand how their nutritional advice affects the health conditions of patients.

Community Dietitians

Community dieticians work in health maintenance organizations, home health agencies, and public health clinics. They counsel individuals and groups on nutritional practices geared towards promoting health and preventing diseases. They evaluate the nutrition needs of individuals and develop personalized healthcare plans. Community dieticians in home health agencies provide instruction on grocery shopping and food preparation practices to individuals with special needs, children, and the elderly.

Consultant Dietitians

Consultant dieticians run their own private practices or work under contract with healthcare facilities, wellness programs, supermarkets, sports teams, and other related businesses. Their knowledge is specialized accordingly. For example, if a consulting dietician is working for a sports team, that consultant will know all about how that particular sport affects the nutritional needs of the athletes. Working for a health club, consultants might specialize in weight loss or nutrition for productive workouts performance. Working for a supermarket, a consultant will know more about how to market nutritionally beneficial food in an appealing way.

One very specialized area of nutritional consultation is at the offices of plastic surgeons. Many people get plastic surgery to improve the way their body looks. Nutritionists help patients develop healthy eating plans post-surgery to keep their bodies looking the way they want them to.

Consultant dieticians may also provide expertise in sanitation, safety procedures, menu development, budgeting, and planning for food service managers in institutions, and restaurant and hotel chains.

On a daily basis, community and consultant dieticians generally perform the following duties:

New patient intake

This usually involves a discussion of health history, an evaluation of current nutritional condition, and goals for improved wellness. Patients may be weighed and/or measured to determine their current condition. The initial consultation may also include a discussion of the social and emotional components of the patient's eating habits. Certain dieticians offer a therapeutic aspect of their services in addition to nutritional advice. This is especially true in the cases of patients with eating disorders.

Sessions with ongoing patients

Dieticians meet with current patients to check on their progress and provide guidance on how to proceed.

Research

Research includes reading well-established books, new books on cutting-edge ideas, internet articles, and nutrition journals. Keeping up to date on the latest nutritional advancements is important for community dieticians because their customers expect them to know all the current information.

Develop specialized recipe ideas, meal plans, and grocery shopping plans for clients. This may involve reading cook books

Consult with other nutritionists and health personnel

Some nutritionists are employed to help treat patients with eating disorders. These professionals may practice in clinical, community, or consultant settings. Regardless of where they work, they must possess specialized knowledge of the physical and psychological effects of eating disorders. They may sometimes serve as therapists for patients who have disordered relationships with food. Their goal is to help their patients regain health and healthy eating patterns.

Management

Management dieticians work in healthcare facilities, schools, company cafeterias, and prisons. They oversee large-scale meal planning and preparation. Part of their job is budgeting and purchasing food, equipment, and supplies. They also enforce sanitary and safety regulations, and prepare records and reports. In addition, they hire, train, and direct other dieticians and food service workers. Their daily duties may include the following:

Meet with kitchen staff to discuss the day's meal plan

Supervise the preparation of food

Create budget plans for food purchasing

Purchase food and any necessary equipment and supplies

Hire, train, evaluate, and fire food service workers as needed

Marketing

Increased public interest in nutrition has led to job opportunities in other sectors as well. The advertising, marketing, and food manufacturing fields are all employers of nutritionists. In these fields, dieticians analyze foods, prepare literature for distribution, and report on the nutritional content of recipes and issues such as dietary fiber and vitamin supplements. Given their intimate knowledge of how food affects people's health and thinking, nutritionists are well suited to designing food advertisements.

Countless magazines and websites include articles on nutrition. Almost all of these articles are written by nutritionists who are savvy enough to get their opinions in print. Popular television programs often invite nutritionists onto their show to give nutritional advice. Those nutritionists include public speaking and travel in their job duties.

The number of people "on a diet" at any given time in the United States is astounding. Diet books are top sellers, and there seems to be no limit to the number being published. This is in part because there are so many different types of recommended diets, but it is mostly due to the public's constant desire to find the quick and easy solution to weight loss problems. Once dieticians prove that their nutrition philosophy can be effective, they can write books and feel confident that they will sell.

Most people have to settle for reading books and magazines. Movie stars, politicians, and other people in the media spotlight have the luxury of hiring nutritionists to develop personalized eating plans for them. Some even have a nutritionist on staff or living in their home. The nutritionist often collaborates with the client's kitchen staff and personal trainer. It is not unusual for such high level nutritionists to enter the media spotlight themselves, especially if they are credited with helping their employer get in shape or overcome some health problem.

Teaching

Many nutritionists are employed by colleges and universities to teach and conduct research. Making a career of nutrition is becoming more and more popular, which means there is a growing need for professionals who can teach nutrition as a field of study. Colleges and universities across the country offer classes in nutrition. Nutrition professors are often engaged in research. In a regular workweek, a nutrition professor can expect to perform the following duties:

Prepare lesson plans for the week's classes.

Teach. Classes may be conducted as large lectures, small seminars, or laboratory research.

Hold office hours. All professors are expected to make time available for students to visit outside of class and ask questions.

Read and grade student work. Some professors may have teaching assistants to help them with this aspect of the job, but almost all professors have some grading to do.

Conduct research.

At large research universities in particular, this may be the most important part of the job. Research includes reading and experimenting. Experiments on the chemical content of food may be conducted in a science laboratory, while experiments on the behavioral aspect of eating patterns may be conducted in public areas such as schools. Behavioral experiments are often long term studies based on careful observation.

Publish

Professors who publish their research in scholarly journals are the ones most likely to land the best jobs and the highest pay. Nutrition is a field that relies on new research findings. Colleges and universities expect their nutrition professors to publish reports on their experimental findings.

Some nutritionists may also work in high schools as home economics or nutrition teachers, or in middle and elementary school to teach basic nutrition. In those cases they are not expected to conduct research like those teaching at the university level. If they are teaching for a public school, their curriculum will most likely be established by the school. At schools with enough resources, nutrition classes may include cooking.

An important part of the job for all types of nutritionists is to eat well and stay fit. Nobody is going to trust a nutritionist who doesn't look healthy. This is truly a field in which professionals must follow their own advice.

PROFESSIONALS WORKING IN THE FIELD TELL THEIR OWN STORIES

I Am a Sports Dietitian

"I am in a really challenging and exciting field, working with high level athletes. It is a specialty that first requires education in clinical dietetics to be able to treat any clinical issues that may arise. Then, through work experience and studies focused on sports nutrition, you prepare to get certification in sports dietetics. The premier professional sports nutrition accreditation is Certified Specialist in Sports Dietetics (CSSD) from Sports, Cardiovascular, and Wellness Nutrition (SCAN), a specialized practice group of the American Dietetic Association.

There is still an element of science in this specialty, but the majority of the work I do is consulting and counseling. Classes like biochemistry can be tough to get through, but good communications skills are just as important in my daily work. The most technical things I do are perform anthropometry testing (human body measurements) and dietary analysis. Most of my time is spent advising individuals and lecturing small groups on optimal eating patterns, nutrient adequacy, and the timing of carbs/protein intake during each training stage. Of course, I am always on the lookout for medical issues such as diabetes, anemia, eating disorders, and food allergies that may need treatment.

Without a doubt, the best thing about this career is getting to work with highly motivated athletes. I feel a real sense of pride and accomplishment when my clients achieve their goals. These days, there is such a minute difference between winning and losing. Yet a simple thing like eating the right food at the right time can give athletes the competitive edge they need to come out on top.

The main challenge in this specialty is finding a good sports dietitian job. You need to cultivate the right contacts any way you can. A good way to do that is to start helping out with a local sports team and working your way up from there. It doesn't matter if you don't get paid. The investment in your future is well worth the effort. Make a name for yourself and with a bit of luck, you could even end up working with a major sports team.

My advice for any aspiring sports dietitian is to get some work experience any way you can. Employers like to see prospects with good credentials. They also respond to those who are passionate about sports nutrition and are using their knowledge to help athletes succeed. Just as the general public has become more aware of the importance of nutrition, so have coaches and fitness staff of sports teams. The benefits of having a specialist sports dietitian working with their athletes are well documented now. That's good because it's creating a growing demand for qualified sports dietitians.

You should also be ready and willing to follow changes in the field. You can't just rely on what you learned in school. You will need to keep up with current trends, monitor the media and scientific journals, and network with other dietitians to learn the latest developments and the emerging research.

I love my job! It is a great feeling making a positive impact on athletes' performance and everyday lives."

I Am a Corporate Food Consultant

"My career has gone from micro to macro. I started out the way so many dietitians do, working one-on-one with individual clients while slowly building a private practice. There were times when I wondered if this was the right profession for me. I didn't feel I was having any impact. It was upsetting to see children getting Type II diabetes, and obese adults eating more French fries than any other vegetable.

One day, while I was lamenting my frustration, a colleague pointed out the obvious – that our profession offers many opportunities. If I didn't feel satisfied with what I was doing, there were plenty of other ways to apply my knowledge and passion. I could get out of clinical work and go into teaching, write professional books or mentor dietitians in private practice, or lecture to dietetic associations. I could go into media work, and educate millions of people on television. I could advise the government on how to help people eat better.

After considering all the options, I determined that I could make the biggest impact as a consultant in the food industry. I now advise food companies on products they can offer consumers. I may not have a seat in the board room, but it feels like a very powerful position to me.

This is an exciting time to be a nutrition professional. How very fortunate we are that we have never seen pellagra or beri beri! We have the safest and most abundant food supply in history. The average local grocery store offers 20,000 foods and most people can afford to choose what they eat. All they need is good information and food products that support healthy choices.

I would encourage anyone who is passionate about food, nutrition, and health to consider this career. I entered this field because I care. The more I learned, the more excited I got about the work I'm doing. Researchers learn more each day about how nutrients protect against disease. My job is to take those new discoveries and make them easily accessible to anyone shopping for dinner. It takes time and patience for my scientific advice to show up on a grocery store shelf, but I am always mindful of the progress that has been made."

PERSONAL QUALIFICATIONS

SUCCESSFUL PROFESSIONALS IN THIS FIELD ARE ABSOLUTELY PASSIONATE ABOUT FOOD AND ITS effects on the body. There are many battles to be fought as a nutritionist. It's not always easy to convince people to change their eating habits. Because there are so many different nutritional philosophies, you must be zealous enough about your own school of thought to keep learning about it, revising it as needed, defending it, and promoting it.

Nutritionists and dietitians must be detail oriented and good with numbers. Preparing meal plans for schools, writing up grocery shopping lists for families, and calculating the calories in recipes are just a few examples of work duties that utilize those skills.

Unless you are engaged primarily with research, you should be a people person. Clinical dietitians working in hospitals are constantly interacting with patients and physicians. Community and consultant dietitians counsel individuals and groups. Management dietitians oversee other staff. Dietitians in schools and universities spend time teaching students and meeting with other faculty. If you're not excited about working directly with people, research may be the best option for you in this career.

In the United States especially, eating can be a very sensitive subject. Eating patterns vary depending on a variety of factors, including region, socioeconomic status, family traditions, and education level. Major food corporations spend huge amounts of money on advertising to influence what people eat. Even the government plays a part by subsidizing certain products. You must take into account all the factors affecting your clients. This requires a thorough knowledge of the food industry, but also communications skills to get the necessary information from the client, and to advise in a non-threatening way. Some nutritionists and dietitians even play the role of a therapist to clients with particularly troubled relationships to food. Empathy and good listening skills are essential to this aspect of the practice.

Writing skills can go a long way in this profession. Many nutritionists and dietitians write articles for journals and magazines, while some even publish their own books. Writing is a way of promoting your philosophy and attracting new clients. Knowing the science isn't enough in this career, you have to be able to communicate it in an appealing manner as well.

Marketing is an important aspect of being a nutritionist or dietitian, especially if you run a private practice. The first step in any marketing plan is to keep yourself fit and healthy. Clients won't be inspired by a so-called nutrition expert who looks unhealthy. Promoting your work through writing is a good idea, as are advertisements, seminars, and workshops. Strong public speaking skills are a must.

New research is constantly coming out that revises, updates, and expands the nutrition field. To keep up with it all, you must have an inquisitive mind. If you're the type of person who wants to learn one methodology and stick with it for the rest of your career, you may get left behind. It is those nutritionists and dietitians who read, write, and attend conferences about nutrition that can truly excel in this field.

ATTRACTIVE FEATURES

ONE OF THE BEST THINGS ABOUT this field is that there are so many different ways to apply your knowledge and experience. As a nutritionist or dietitian, you can work in a wide range of settings, from schools to hospitals to universities, prisons, supermarket chains – from private practices to community health centers. There are also many different schools of nutritional thought. Whether you believe in the Atkins diet or veganism, there is a place for you in this career.

Increasing public awareness of nutrition has brought nutritionists and dietitians into the spotlight. It is commonplace to see nutritionists speaking on talk shows, and read articles about nutrition they write in the newspaper. Nutritionists and dietitians are at the forefront of the fight to decrease the rates of obesity and diseases such as diabetes in this country. You can expect positive recognition, whether it is from individual clients who have succeeded in losing weight, parents whose children are eating healthier school lunches, or hospital patients whose health has improved as a result of dietary changes. You have the satisfaction of knowing that you are improving people's health and quality of life on a daily basis.

Unlike doctors, nutritionists and dietitians don't have to deal with the high-risk, high-stress situations of patients in life or death conditions. Instead, you provide preventative and treatment care to improve patients' health over the long-term. This means that your work is very rewarding without much pressure.

Continually meeting new people is a fundamental part of this field. Nutritionists and dietitians of all sorts are constantly working with new clients, students, and colleagues. This keeps the job interactive and dynamic. Although much of nutrition is science based, that doesn't mean that you will be shut up in a lab doing research all the time.

The work environment is very pleasant. Facilities are typically clean and modern. You can depend on working no more than an ordinary 40-hour workweek, although some of those hours may be on the weekends. If you are self-employed or work as part of a private practice, you can determine your own hours, or work part time. Very few nutritionists and dietitians are required to be on-call. For those who prefer to pursue a part-time career, this field offers plenty of opportunities. In fact, about 20 percent of the nutritionist and dietitian population work part time by choice.

The job outlook is good. The aging population, in particular, has many special nutritional needs. As this segment of the population increases, so does the demand for nutritional professionals. The chances of finding a job are especially good if you have an advanced degree, specialized training, licensure and certification.

One of the best parts of this job is working alongside people who believe in the health-giving powers of food. By becoming a nutritionist or dietitian, you are joining a community based on healing. This is incredibly rewarding for those who believe wholeheartedly in what they do.

UNATTRACTIVE FEATURES

ALTHOUGH THE JOB CAN BE rewarding when you make a positive difference in the health of your clients, it can also be discouraging when you fail. The number of unhealthy patients you see on a daily basis can be overwhelming. Some of them will be reluctant to follow your advice, and may end up never improving. Public schools and prisons are notorious for bad food. Even if you do your best to improve the eating standards, funding can be limited, and you may find that your input isn't making much of a difference.

Nutrition is a vast field with a huge variety of job descriptions. The type of job you are most interested in may not be open when you enter the job market. You may find yourself working in areas that you don't feel passionate about. This is especially true as the nutrition field changes. For example, as hospitals begin switching to outside food services, the jobs for nutritionists and dietitians within hospitals will decline, forcing them to look for jobs in the outside food services sector.

When government funding for public schools, hospitals, community health centers and prisons is cut back, you may find yourself searching for jobs in the private sector. It can be difficult to set up or join a private practice. Attracting new patients takes time. Once you have established a patient base, you will have little freedom to change location.

The research on nutrition is constantly changing. This can be exciting and keep you on your toes, but it can also endanger your credibility. If, for example, you are a proponent of a low-fat diet and research comes out about how important fat is in the diet, your clients may stop trusting you. Often it doesn't matter which theory is correct, but which theory is getting the most publicity. It can get tiring to be constantly defending your philosophy.

In comparison to many other health professions, nutritionists and dietitians are paid relatively modest salaries. The median annual earnings are $55,000, and even with advancement you won't get to a six-figure salary.

The pressure of staying fit and healthy can require your time and energy. Eating well and exercising in accordance with your own philosophy are prerequisites for most nutritionists and dietitians. This can be both expensive and time consuming.

EDUCATION AND TRAINING

THIS IS A CAREER THAT REQUIRES study of dietetics, foods and nutrition, food service systems management, and other areas of knowledge. Most jobs require a bachelor's degree and many employers prefer to employ people with a master's degree.

Educational programs are readily available. In the US, there are 270 bachelor's degree programs and 18 master's degree programs approved by the American Dietetic Association's Commission on Accreditation for Dietetics Education.

The programs include courses in chemistry, biochemistry, physiology, biology, microbiology, institution management, foods, and nutrition. Related and recommended courses include psychology, sociology, communications, business, computer science, mathematics, statistics, and economics. The reason for the diversity of courses is that nutritionists need to prepare for employment in a number of different workplaces.

Many of the colleges and universities that offer bachelor's degrees in dietetics follow the curriculum set by the American Dietetic Association. The curriculum is designed for a four-year degree program. It includes classroom instruction in clinical dietetics with core courses in human nutrition, medical nutrition therapy, experimental foods, quantity food production, and food service organization. Students in such programs are often able to enter directly into a supervised practicum or internship.

Master's degrees often qualify dietitians for research, public health, or advanced clinical positions. A master's degree is a good idea for dietitians who want to advance in their careers, or for people who already hold a bachelor's degree in an unrelated field and want to become a dietitian. Master of Science in Nutrition programs focus on research and clinical methods in dietetics and nutrition. Developmental nutrition, nutritional biochemistry, exercise physiology, metabolism, and research methods are all key points of the course of study. A master's thesis is often required.

Licensure

Currently, 46 states and jurisdictions have laws governing dietetics practice. Of these, 33 require licensure, 12 require statutory certification, and one merely requires registration. Specific requirements vary state by state. Job candidates are expected to understand and fulfill the requirements of the state in which they want to work before sitting for any exam.

Licensure is the strictest form of state regulation. Only people who are licensed can work as nutritionists and dietitians in states that require licensure. The situation is less restrictive in states that require certification. Those states generally limit the use of occupational titles to people who meet certain requirements. This means that individuals without certification can still practice as a nutritionist or dietitian; they are just not allowed to use certain titles.

Registration is the least restrictive form of state regulation in this field. Currently, only California prohibits unregistered nutritionists and dietitians to work in the state.

Certification

The American Dietetic Association awards the Registered Dietitian (RD) credential to those who pass an exam after completing a bachelor's degree at an approved institution in addition to a supervised internship.

The internship can be completed in one of two ways. The first option is to complete a program accredited by the Commission on Dietetic Registration. There are 51 accredited programs that include academic and supervised practice experience. These programs typically last four to five years and effectively combine the bachelor's degree with an internship. The second option is to complete 900 hours of supervised practice experience in one of 243 accredited internships, in addition to the bachelor's degree. These internships generally take place in a healthcare or food service facility.

EARNINGS

THE MEDIAN ANNUAL WAGE OF dietitians and nutritionists is about $55,000. Most earn between $45,000 and $65,000. Overall, earnings can vary widely though. A few earn as little as $35,000 while some earn more than $75,000. As with all professions, salary can vary depending on years in practice, education level, geographic location, facility, and duties. Here are the annual salaries for dietitians in different practice areas as documented by the American Dietetic Association:

Community nutrition
$48,000

Clinical nutrition/acute care
$49,000

Clinical nutrition/ambulatory care
$52,000

Clinical nutrition/long-term care
$54,000

Consultation and business
$60,000

Food and nutrition management
$64,000

Education and research
$66,000

The industries employing the largest number of dietitians and nutritionists pay the following salaries on average:

Special food services
$45,000

Local government
$47,000

Nursing care facilities
$51,000

General medical and surgical hospitals
$51,000

Outpatient care centers
$52,000

It is not unusual for nutritionists and dietitians to be in practice for themselves. These self-employed professionals enjoy the potential of earning considerably more than their salaried colleagues. However, actual earnings depend on marketing and business skills. Earnings also vary by geographic region in accordance with economic demographics – especially for nutritionists and dietitians catering to individual clients. Richer areas often have people who are willing to pay more money to keep up a fit and healthy appearance. Hollywood is one of the best examples of this.

Those who are self-employed must typically supply their own insurance and other benefits. Those employed by health clinics, hospitals, wellness centers, schools, and any other government facility generally receive benefits packages that include health insurance, retirement plans, sick leave, and paid vacation.

OPPORTUNITIES

JOB PROSPECTS FOR NUTRITIONISTS and dietitians are expected to be good for the foreseeable future. Those with an advanced degree, specialized training, or more certifications than the basic ones required by the state will have the best job prospects. Those without a bachelor's degree will face the toughest competition.

The increasing emphasis on disease prevention through the improvement of dietary habits will result in job growth for nutritionists and dietitians. Popular public interest has already had a positive effect on the employment rates for this field. As health education takes on a more prominent role in public schools, this trend is expected to continue. Those working in food service management will reap the most benefits.

A growing and aging population raises demand for nutritional counseling and treatment in hospitals, home healthcare agencies, residential care facilities, community health programs, schools, and prisons. Clinical, community, consultant, and management dietitians will see increased employment opportunities as a result.

Nutritionists and dietitians specializing in certain diseases will have an advantage. The increased public awareness of obesity and diabetes has led Medicare to expand its coverage to include medical nutrition therapy for renal and diabetic patients. The aging population has created an increased demand for nutritionists and dietitians specializing in gerontological nutrition.

Hospitals are expected to continue to employ a large number of dietitians and nutritionists to plan meals and provide medical nutritional therapy. However, they will also continue to contract with outside agencies such as food services. Many are expected to transfer medical nutritional therapy to outpatient care facilities. These changes will slow job growth for those employees working in hospital food services and inpatient facilities. The number of dietitian positions in nursing care facilities is also expected to decline as the facilities turn to outside agencies for food services.

These changes are not bad news for nutritionists and dietitians, however. Employment is expected to grow rapidly with contract providers of food services, in the offices of physicians and other health practitioners, and in outpatient care centers.

Insurance policies are the biggest determinant of demand for nutritional services. Although more insurance plans now cover nutritional therapy services, the extent of coverage can vary greatly between plans. Employment growth can be slowed by limitations on insurance reimbursement for dietetic services. As nutrition therapy is typically not considered an emergency treatment, many clients are unwilling to pay large out-of-pocket expenses, unless they view it as being absolutely necessary.

GETTING STARTED

NUTRITIONISTS AND DIETITIANS HAVE choices to make. There are a variety of different work settings, which makes it important to decide early on in your college career what specific type of work you would like to be doing. All nutrition majors have core requirements, but there are many related courses and electives available. You should choose the classes best suited to your specific field of interest. For example, if you're thinking about a career in food service management, you may want to add marketing and economics classes to your course list.

Research is a great thing to get on your résumé. Take classes that include a laboratory component. Ideally, you should work with a nutrition professor who is publishing research. Getting your name listed as a co-author or laboratory assistant on a published research study is an excellent way to prove that you are committed to the field and ready for higher level work. This is especially true for those nutrition and dietetic students planning on earning a master's degree.

One of the most important factors to consider early on is which state you want to work in. Licensure, certification, and registration requirements vary state by state. You want to make sure that you are preparing for the right requirements. If you want to work in a state that requires certification, you should start looking for internship opportunities to complete the internship requirement. An internship is also one of the best ways to segue into a full-time job.

Ask your professors for ideas on where to look for internships and jobs. Your college career counselor should be able to help you as well. Associations such as the American Dietetic Association and the American Nutrition Association are also good resources. They provide lists of job and internship openings in addition to information about the field. You can also use employment agencies that specialize in finding nutrition and dietetic jobs. Just make sure that when you apply anywhere that your résumé is polished and ready.

As with most professions, letters of recommendation are key to landing your first job. You should build connections with professors early on so that when the time comes for them to write you a recommendation, they will remember what it is they like about you.

Nutrition and dietetics is an interconnected field. You may find someday down the line that a fellow classmate is working somewhere where you would like to get a job. It is important in college to treat your classmates as colleagues, not competitors. If you end up applying to one of them for a job in the future, you want them to feel happy to work with you.

ASSOCIATIONS

■ **American Dietetic Association**
http://www.eatright.org

■ **The International & American Associations of Clinical Nutritionists (IAACN)**
http://www.iaacn.org

■ **The National Association of Nutrition Professionals (NANP)**
http://www.nanp.org

■ **The American Nutrition Association**
http://americannutritionassociation.org

■ **Collegiate & Professional Sports Dietitians Association**
http://www.sportsrd.org

■ **Sports, Cardiovascular, and Wellness Nutrition**
http://www.scandpg.org

PERIODICALS

■ **Today's Dietician**
http://www.todaysdietitian.com

■ **Nutritionist World**
http://www.nutritionist-world.com

■ **Today's Diet and Nutrition**
http://www.tdn-digital.com

WEBSITES

■ **Dietetics Online**
http://www.dietetics.com

■ **Food Science and Human Nutrition (FSHN) Club**
http://uffshnclub.webs.com

■ **Utah State University,**
School of Agriculture
http://ndfs.usu.edu/dietetics

■ **Commission on Dietetic Registration (CDR)**
http://www.cdrnet.org

■ **Allen Foundation**
https://www.allenfoundation.org

■ **Nutrition That Works**
www.consultantdietitians.com

■ **Consultant Dietitians in Health Care Facilities**
www.healthboard.com/websites
/Detailed/28918.html

Copyright 2015

Institute For Career Research

Website www.careers-internet.org

For information on other Careers Reports please contact

service@careers-internet.org

www.ingramcontent.com/pod-product-compliance
Lightning Source LLC
Chambersburg PA
CBHW070938290526
45795CB00003B/1061